EAR CANDLING MADE SIMPLE

A STEP BY STEP GUIDE
AND INSTRUCTIONS ON
EAR CANDLING AND IT'S
EFFECTS

CAMILLA LOOMIS

Table of Contents

CHAPTER ONE

CANDLEMASS EAR WAX

Is it ok to use candles in your ears?

Ear candling, in which a lit candle is placed in a person's ear, is an unsafe and unproven practice. The candle's warmth is meant to remove wax and other debris from the ear.

Ear candling advocates claim the practice can help with

everything from earwax buildups to cancer.

In this article, we'll define ear candling, talk about its safety, and examine any potential drawbacks.

So, what exactly is ear candling?

Coning, or ear candling, is a complementary medicine practiced by some to remove earwax and other debris from the middle ear.

The standard ear candle is a hollow, tapered cylinder that

measures about 10 inches in length. The wide end is where they are lit.

Typically, they are crafted from fabric that has been drenched in a wax or wax-like substance (such as paraffin and beeswax).

Ear candling entails placing a candle in a patient's ear while they are lying on their side. A square or circle of paper, tin foil, or plastic is used as a cover to keep the hot wax off the face, neck, and hair.

After making sure both the candle and its covering are in place, the latter is lit for ten to twenty minutes. In this method, wax does not enter the ear canal.

Ear candling goes by a few different names.

- Coning of the ear canal
- Auricular or Thermal Heat Therapy
- Chandelier or cone treatment

Why is this idea being put forth, and what are its potential advantages?

When you or your child is having ear trouble, it's important to see a doctor.

Ear candling has not been shown to have any positive effects in clinical trials. Ear candling continues to be promoted by its proponents and manufacturers as having numerous advantages. Unsubstantiated claims have been made by some manufacturers, including that their products can aid in the treatment of certain forms of cancer.

Ear candling may have additional benefits, including but not limited to the following:

Cleaning the ear canal of wax, bacteria, and other debris

The Management of Sinus Infections

It can help with hearing and even reverse hearing loss.

- soothing throat pain

The management of respiratory illnesses

This includes, but is not limited to:

Increased focus and clarity of thought

Blood purification

Intensifying lymphatic flow

- reducing eye strain and enhancing clarity of vision

Reducing the discomfort of TMDs and other jaw problems

- alleviating nervousness and anxiety

Among its benefits is a diminished sensation of dizziness.

Many people who advocate for the use of ear candles state that the suction created by the candle's heat is the primary benefit. With the help of this suction, ear wax and other debris can be removed from the ear.

These assertions are illogical, and there is no scientific proof that ear candles have the purported benefits.

Earwax is a self-cleaning, lubricating, and antibacterial substance for the ear canal, despite the fact that many people dislike it. Ears of people who don't produce enough earwax tend to get dry and itchy.

The removal of earwax is a natural occurrence that occurs when you chew or swallow.

Earwax dries and falls out of the ear once it has left the ear canal.

Wax can accumulate in the ear canal. Ear wax becomes more embedded in the canal when a person repeatedly pushes it deeper with their finger. Earwax can be caused by anything inserted into the ear, from cotton swabs to paper clips.

If your ears are blocked by wax, you might experience the following symptoms:

- discomfort in the ear

• ringing in the ears (also known as tinnitus)

Partial deafness

• Earwax buildup

Ears that stink

• ear tingling

• an earache, or the sensation that one's ear canal is blocked

Have we established that it is safe to do so?

The FDA has issued a warning that ear candling should not be practiced for safety reasons. Since early 2010, they have been advising the public to avoid the method and any associated products.

Ear candling carries a high risk of injury and has no verified health benefits.

A study conducted in 2016 followed a 16-year-old boy who used ear candling to treat his allergies and found that the practice caused him pain and impaired his hearing. Candle stubs and other bits of wax were lodged in his eardrum, and a doctor had to clean them out.

The FDA is concerned about the potential danger ear candling poses to the public. They have seized products from "coning practitioners" and "ear candle retailers" and issued warnings to the former.

Possible adverse effects

Pin ItThe use of an open flame and molten wax in an ear candle presents several safety hazards.

Major health authorities, including the Food and Drug Administration (FDA), have been sounding the alarm about the risks associated with ear candles for years.

Potential dangers and negative effects could include:

• being burned by hot wax or ash in the face, neck, eardrum, middle ear, or ear canal

A few examples are: • lighting a fire

• eardrum perforation

Example: plugging your ears with candle wax

- bleeding
- acquiring subsequent infections

Feeling a temporary loss of hearing

obtaining swimmer's ear, also known as otitis externa

triggering middle ear dysfunction

A child's natural tendency to move around during the procedure increases the likelihood that some of the hot wax or ash will escape the covering and cause injury.

Similarly, the ear canals of children are noticeably smaller than those of adults. Because of this, they are more likely to become clogged.

It's possible that people with ear infections or other conditions that need medical attention would let them get worse if they tried ear candling first.

CHAPTER TWO

The proper technique for extracting an earwig

Many people would freak out if they thought a bug was scurrying around in their ear. It's not common, but it is possible for a bug to get inside your ear and stay there for a while.

The bug can enter the ear through a few different entry points. It could sneak in while they slept, or it could fly into their ear while they were outside.

Even if an insect makes it into the ear, it might not survive for long. On the other hand, there is always a chance that it will manage to stay alive and keep on moving.

Even though ear bugs usually don't cause any serious issues, they can occasionally develop into something more serious. However risky it may be, most people would rather have the bug out of their ear as soon as possible.

The telltale signs of an earworm Sometimes people get bugs in their ears and don't even realize it until they start experiencing symptoms. If you have a bug in your ear, you're probably experiencing some pain or discomfort.

Several cranial nerves connect the outer ear and the outer side of the eardrum to the brain. These nerves can be triggered by something as simple as a bug.

Possible causes of unusual aural sensations include the insect's continued existence and the insect's potential to be actively crawling or buzzing.

Depending on the bug, it may also sting or bite repeatedly as it is stuck in the ear, which can be excruciating.

There may be other signs of an ear infection, such as:

- a stuffed-out sensation in the ear

- swelling

Ear discharges of blood or pus

Hearing loss

How to Carefully Extract an Insect

The key to successfully removing a bug from your ear or the ear of another person is to remain calm.

However unsettling it may be to have a bug in one's ear, worrying about it will only make matters worse.

To get rid of an earwig, do the following:

To remove the bug, tilt your head to the side where it is lodged and shake your head gently. Do not cause further damage by hitting your ear.

If the insect is still alive, you can try to suffocate it by pouring a very small amount of vegetable oil into its ear.

- Use warm water to flush the bug out of your ear if it is dead.

Don't insert foreign objects like tweezers or cotton swabs into your ear canal. These factors may increase the bug's proximity to the eardrum, increasing the risk of injury or even deafness.

If your child has a history of ear problems, such as frequent infections, tympanostomy tubes, or a perforated eardrum, it is best to get medical help rather than trying to remove the bug yourself.

Precautions

Do not insert anything, including a cotton swab or other probing device, into the ear canal when trying to remove a bug from the ear at home.

Forcing an insect deeper into the ear canal by inserting a sharp object can have devastating consequences.

Attempts by an untrained person to remove an object from someone's ear have been linked to an increased risk of a number of complications, according to the study's authors.

A ruptured eardrum is one of the potential complications that can arise from cuts and bruises to the external ear canal.

Reasons to Visit the Doctor

When an ear bug cannot be removed at home, prompt medical attention is necessary to avoid further complications.

Leaving an insect in the ear can increase the risk of infection and even a perforated eardrum from repeated stinging and scratching. Also possible is infection.

The otoscope allows the doctor to examine the ear canal from the outside.

Mineral or olive oil is typically used to kill the insect before it is flushed out of the ear with sterile water.

If they are unable to flush it out, they may attempt to grab it with tiny forceps.

In most cases, a local anesthetic is all that's needed to keep the patient still and calm during the bug removal procedure.

Only 13.6% of people in one study who had something stuck in their ear required general anesthesia for removal.

With or without the use of local anesthesia, doctors were able to successfully remove the foreign body in 86.4% of cases using forceps, suction, a probe, a fine hook, or an ear syringe.

Once the bug has been removed, the pain and other symptoms will typically disappear as well. Inflammation caused by stings or scratches can last for several days.

Antibiotics are useful for the prevention of infections, but they may be required in some cases.

Prevention

People can't completely eliminate the possibility of an insect crawling into their ear, but they can take some precautions to lessen the odds. Some examples are:

- protecting yourself from mosquitoes and other biting insects whenever you're out in the country

- putting in earplugs before going camping

- maintaining a spotless house to lessen the possibility of pests

It is often possible to get rid of a bug that has gotten into your ear with some common household items. You should see a doctor immediately if these don't help.

The proper technique for removing impacted earwax

Care Options: Professional and Natural

Ear Candling

- Safety

Earwax Removal Kit Instructions

- Symptoms

- Prevention

Visiting a Medical Practitioner

CHAPTER THREE

Cerumen, or earwax, is a naturally occurring substance that helps keep the ears clean and dry. It aids in the elimination of ear wax, dirt, hair, and other debris.

Cleaning out your ear canal with earwax once in a while can reduce the chance of infection and alleviate any discomfort or itching you might be experiencing. It also helps lessen the discomfort that can result from water getting into the ear canal.

But sometimes the body produces too much earwax, and it becomes a problem when it blocks the ear canal.

Cotton swabs aren't the best choice for ear cleaning because they can actually cause more earwax to be pushed deeper into the ear canal, leading to a blockage. Using a hearing aid can increase the risk of this happening.

A cerumen impaction is the medical term for an earwax blockage, and it is usually treated at home with common remedies.

CHAPTER FOUR

Medications and natural cures

A buildup of earwax can be dealt with in a number of ways at home.

Water with a little bit of bleach added to it, or hydrogen peroxide

A cotton ball dipped in hydrogen peroxide is a common home remedy for earwax buildup. Some people use hydrogen peroxide as an antiseptic because it is widely available and considered to be a reliable source of information. A sterile eyedropper can also be used to administer the solution directly into the ear canal.

Tilting the head so that the affected ear faces upward for a few minutes is recommended. The fluid can then slowly trickle down into the ear canal and reach the obstruction.

After waiting a few minutes, you can clear out any remaining fluid or earwax by tilting your head in the opposite direction.

Hydrogen peroxide should be applied to earwax about 30 minutes before ear irrigation, as suggested by one study. Earwax can be more easily removed with water irrigation after being softened by the solution.

Pure hydrogen peroxide solutions, or drops made from them, should be used with caution. Hydrogen peroxide can irritate the skin, even when used in the low concentrations found in common household products. The skin can be burned if exposed to concentrations of 10% or higher.

Anyone experiencing irritation should stop using the product immediately and contact their doctor if their condition worsens.

Hydrogen peroxide should only be used if the eardrum has not been punctured. Pain is experienced if the eardrum is perforated or ear tubes have been placed.

Toy syringe with rubber ball

Using a rubber ball syringe and hot water is another option. When using a syringe, the affected ear should be facing upward while warm water is slowly dripped into the ear canal.

One must take care not to force water into one's ear canal, as this can lead to vertigo. The water temperature needs to be just right.

The next step is to tilt the head the other way after a minute to allow the fluid and earwax to drain. A slight tug on the ear can help the water drain out.

It's possible that this will need to be done more than once. No one with an ear injury, such as a perforated eardrum, should try this. Regular sufferers of swimmer's ear should avoid this method.

Hearing Loss

Ear drops for removing earwax buildup can be bought without a prescription at most pharmacies or online. Earwax softening solutions can either be water- or oil-based. Carbamide peroxide, which is chemically related to hydrogen peroxide, is frequently included in these products.

A person using an over-the-counter remedy must adhere to the directions printed on the product's container. The affected ear will need to have the solution applied to it twice daily for several days until the ear canal is clear.

A combination of the ear drops and the warm water and rubber syringe to flush or irrigate the ear may be necessary if the earwax is not removed entirely by the ear drops. After 4 days, a person should consult a doctor about the issue.

Alternatives to commercial drugs

It is possible to apply other substances with an eyedropper as well. Other products that can help clear wax, according to a 2018 article, are:

Baby oil

- saline

- oil derived from almonds, arches, or camphor that has been refined

Oils of Almond or Mineral

10 percent sodium bicarbonate

- glycerin

- 2.5% acetic acid

Cotton swabs, ear candling, and the use of olive oil in the form of drops or sprays are all things that are discouraged in the same article.

Again, the affected ear should be held at an upward angle while one or two drops are applied; after a few minutes, the head should be tilted in the opposite direction to allow the fluid to drain. No one should put anything in their ear unless their eardrum is not only intact but also has been cleared by a doctor.

The question is whether or not ear candles are appropriate.

Ear candles are not effective in clearing impacted ear canals, so they should be avoided.

Ear coning, or thermal-auricular therapy, is another name for using ear candles. To do this, one dips a hollow fabric cone into wax or paraffin, places it in the ear of a supine person, and lights it. A paper plate can catch any dripping wax and prevent it from touching the skin.

Ear candling is thought to work by creating suction, which then removes the earwax.

A study from 2016 suggests that ear candling is not a good idea, and that there are safer ways to get rid of earwax. The Food and Drug Administration (FDA) has taken several ear candle products off the market due to safety concerns, and the American Academy of Otolaryngology-Head and Neck Surgery Foundation also advises against their use.

Ear candles are not a good idea because there are better and safer ways to remove earwax buildup.

Have we established that it is safe to do so?

When done correctly, with the help of a home kit or a doctor's advice, earwax removal at home is safe.

However, there are a few exceptions to the rule that say not everyone can safely remove earwax at home. However, there are some people who should not use any home remedies or over-the-counter kits from Trusted Source, and those people are:

Those who: • are unable to maintain a standard sitting position

• have something lodged in your ear

have inner ear problems or a history of ear surgery

Have a perforated ear drum

• contract swimmer's ear

have a severe case of swimmer's ear

have a family history of middle ear disease

radiation exposure

No one should try to remove earwax on their own if they have any doubts about whether or not they should.

CHAPTER FIVE

Removal of Earwax: A Step-by-Step Guide

The effectiveness of earwax removal kits and irrigation systems varies slightly from one model to the next, and even within a single model. Before using the kit, the patient should consult with his or her doctor and follow all of the directions on the package and the instructions provided by the medical professional.

Using irrigation or a home kit system, these are the typical steps a person will take to remove earwax in 2021, as reported by a reputable article:

1.

Finding a comfortable chair to sit upright in, tilting the head to one side, and then placing a few drops of warm water, saline, hydrogen peroxide, or the solution provided in the kit into the ear is the recommended method.

2.

They should then take 15 to 30 minutes to sit with their head cocked to one side.

3.

Ear wax should be soaked in the solution, and then the ear should be sucked into the bulb or flushed with the provided device.

4.

As soon as they're done, they need to dry off the area around them.

Problems call for an immediate trip to the doctor.

Symptoms

Blockage of the ear canal by earwax typically causes temporary deafness or difficulty hearing, according to a reliable source. Worry not; normal hearing should resume after the obstruction is removed.

Some additional symptoms could be:

an aural migraine or earache

- ringing in the ears, also known as tinnitus

- dizziness

- a stuffed-out sensation in the ear

Prevention

It's not a good idea to stick cotton swabs or anything else in your ear to clean it because it could lead to an earwax blockage or make an existing one worse. Why? Because the foreign bodies cause the earwax to be pushed deeper into the ear canal.

Sticking objects into one's ear canal can cause a buildup of earwax and should be avoided. Despite its unattractive appearance, earwax rarely requires removal. Ears can naturally expel most wax on their own.

People can get safe relief from excessive earwax buildup by using over-the-counter ear drops.

Earwax blockages can also be avoided by regularly putting drops of a solution meant to soften earwax into one's ears. Shoppers have a wide selection of products to choose from when shopping online.

Drops for removing earwax

Petroleum mineral

* Hydrogen peroxide

Although ear irrigation can help prevent earwax buildups, it is usually reserved for use when an actual blockage has occurred.

In no circumstances should an adult irrigate a child's ears without first consulting with a medical professional.

Reasons to Visit the Doctor

The majority of earwax blockages are easily remedied by the patient themselves. The ear canal and eardrum, however, are sensitive, so it may be best to have a doctor remove earwax.

Ear pain that is severe or accompanied by bleeding or drainage from the ear indicates a more serious problem and warrants medical attention.

It is recommended that anyone worried about an infant or young child's impacted cerumen schedule an appointment with a pediatrician. They can evaluate the child's hearing and make treatment suggestions.

A doctor can use instruments designed specifically for the ear to remove the obstruction.

If symptoms persist or worsen despite at-home care, medical

attention may be warranted after a few days.

www.ingramcontent.com/pod-product-compliance
Lightning Source LLC
La Vergne TN
LVHW010505160826
845677LV00012B/2659

* 9 7 9 8 8 4 7 0 8 3 3 2 4 *